Embrace It:

Loving Life with Vitiligo

Cynthia K. Robertson, MS

Embrace It: Loving Life with Vitiligo

ISBN (979-8-9898507-6-1)

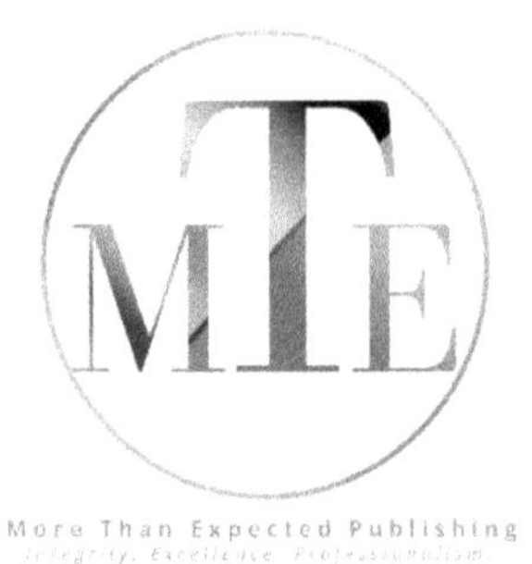

MTE Publishing
mtepublishing.com

Table of Contents

Acknowledgements & Encouragement

This book was written to provide encouragement as I share my journey living with vitiligo. I encourage those who do not have the model body image on the outside as most of the world. This includes those with skin disorders such as vitiligo, alopecia, severe acne, and those who are seen as being too thick, thin, smaller, bigger, missing body parts, teeth, wear glasses or whatever the case may be.

This literary work would not be possible if it weren't for people in my life who invested in me, encouraged me, laughed with me, cried with mec., and supported me. I was once a very private person who would only share when I wanted to and only with those I wanted to share with.

In 2020 my life as I knew it changed and although I toiled for months, I finally realized that my story was more than skin deep! My life can be an inspiration and blessing to those with the auto immune disorder of vitiligo similar to mine.

I thank my parents Roosevelt Branch and Ella Kelley Branch Baskin (who are both deceased) for instilling confidence, determination, knowledge, and faith within me. These personal attributes have empowered me tremendously!

I thank my sons Johnny A. Robertson and Chance D. Robertson for loving their "momma" unconditionally regardless of the public view of my outer self. To my late brother Roy Chet, (who lovingly calls me Ms. Daisy)… Your words, *"When a man looks at you, he will see why God chose you!"* I am thankful to my sisters Rosetta Branch Haines and Latoya Branch; I never worry because I know you two will always have my front and my back! Especially, when people are openly judgmental about my vitiligo, Ella's Angels to *my* rescue.

Finally, to **"MY FRIEND,"** you know who you are. You pushed me and when I didn't move fast enough and then you pushed me again! You knew my potential when I first mentioned writing about vitiligo. You encouraged me to show the world MY greatness. No matter where life takes us, we will remain okay with our 35 plus years friendship. I am forever grateful.

Chapter 1

The Beginning: Snaggle Tooth & Changing Colors

Beauty begins the moment we EMBRACE ourselves.
~Cynthia K. Robertson

My skin revealed signs of depigmentation at the intuitive age of seven. The discoloration initially surfaced around my eyes and mouth… So, my skin was changing colors, and I lost my baby teeth simultaneously. Surprisingly, I was not self-conscious at all. However, my parents didn't know what my condition was, and they began taking me to several doctors… Unfortunately, they were not familiar with dermatological conditions, especially within the African American community.

My father was determined to find a treatment for the sudden changes to my skin. We traveled monthly to a doctor in Ocala, Florida and tried every treatment that was available during this time. Lovingly, my father *always* affirmed me. Therefore,I felt and believed that I was beautiful because my daddy said so! My father knew there were people in the world that were not always kind when they encountered people that were different. I remained happy and confident no matter what anyone said! Their words didn't matter because I didn't believe them! These trips gave me the most unforgettable memories of my father. After every appointment, daddy happily bought me the "treat" of my choice! I was *daddy's girl…* And if I wanted it, *Daddy, got it!*

A dermatologist told my father that my skin discoloration was due to a vitamin deficiency. However, its origin and treatment were unknown. I was given vitamins and a cream to apply to my skin daily and was cautioned to avoid the sun as much as possible! My father and I traveled back and forth to numerous doctors, and we tried countless skincare products until my adolescent years.

Relentlessly, white-colored patches continued to surface around my eyes, and on my fingertips. The progression of my skin re-pigmenting seemed slower than molasses. I couldn't foresee my skin being "*normal*" again. Whether my eyeglasses were on or off, I couldn't DENY my reflection, so I EMBRACED it!

During puberty my body changed and so did the appearance of my skin. The discoloration increased tremendously, specifically on my elbows, knees, and feet. These changes seemingly appeared *overnight*! I was astonished by how rapidly Vitiligo transformed my identity.

As I grew older, additional methods of treatment became available. PUVA treatments stand out in my mind. The treatment consisted of taking a drug PSORALEN (P) and then exposing the skin to long-wave ultra- violet light to stimulate pigment growth. These treatments were conducted three times a week. However, it caused a sunburn appearance and produced little to no dark freckles that were medically termed as *islands*.

The purpose of the island appearance was to create dark spots on my skin that would blend and eventually cover a large area of my discolored skin. Being the knowledge-seeker I am, I researched vitiligo. I needed to understand Vitiligo because we were now walking hand in hand - *daily*.

I read several articles and medical journals that stated that prescribed exposure of UV light and direct sunlight exposure could cause skin cancer. I hadn't been taught to wear sunscreen when I was outside… I didn't know many Black folks who did. So, I was extremely leery of continuing the PUVA treatments and shortly after I discontinued it. I'd rather have my dalmatian looking skin than increase my chances of getting cancer. Besides, the restoration of fully melanated skin was minimal to none.

Thankfully, I was not emotionally affected by my skin changing colors. My immediate and extended family were/are extremely supportive. They never made me feel as if I was different from anyone else in our family.

Our dedication, loyalty, and commitment to each other was always positive and consistent. There have been several instances when people blatantly stared at me when I was in public. Some of them even had the audacity to ask my parents or other family members if I had been in a fire.

Surprisingly (at the time), adults were more verbal and critical of my appearance than young children. Adults didn't say the darndest things, the things they said were ignorantly inconsiderate. Some asked if they could touch me. Other folks asked if the discoloration hurt. Church folks thought I had leprosy that is spoken of in the bible.

After being bombarded with questions and statements, that "othered" me, I knew at that very moment… I wanted to be an advocate for those who have been gifted with Vitiligo and educate my community and possibly the world about it!

In the early 1960's (my childhood years), skin disorders among African Americans were not as noticeable or prevalent as they are today! As a child, I was unaware that people of all ethnicities and nationalities had vitiligo *too*. Sadly, many of them felt more comfortable hiding their appearance from the public.

Quite frequently, because I chose to embrace my skin, people didn't shy away from asking me about my uniquely beautiful appearance.

During the summer, because I wasn't accustomed to wearing sunscreen, my skin was always inflamed and irritated with blistering and peeling. I was fascinated at how my peeling BROWN skin would shed and produce a WHITE appearance.

Although I was the only one with vitiligo among my siblings, I was not treated differently in any capacity by my family or my extended support system. My neighborhood friends never questioned the changes of my skin, nor did they taunt me or attempt to embarrass me. They accepted and loved my unique beauty.

I was always supported and protected. When newcomers to our neighborhood questioned the lightness around my eyes and fingers, my neighborhood riders immediately responded, "That's how God made her." Then we returned to playing without missing a beat!

I genuinely loved and accepted MY skin! I always believed I was beautiful from the inside out… When people saw me, they instantly saw that my beauty was skin deep!

My middle and high school experiences paled in comparison to elementary school. I was introduced to new people with different mindsets. They'd never known or seen anyone with Vitiligo. I realized my skin disorder may have been a culture shock to them, but it was an everyday grind for me. I never felt ashamed of my outer appearance, nor did I shy away from school or school activities. I participated in several extracurricular activities in school. I was also a cheerleader. My natural tenaciousness and ingrained confidence caused me to never shy away from accomplishing what I desired. Like I said, I embraced me even if no one else did, I fell in love with myself!

Reflect & Embrace It:

Reflection is a necessary practice for those who desire TO LOVE & EMBRACE themselves completely… DO this now, you're worth it!

Living life with an autoimmune disorder that changes your outer appearance can be complex and rewarding. The lessons learned from those who don't understand the changes that are quickly and quietly taking place within your body *will* do one of two things: create self-awareness and build self-confidence OR create self-doubt.

REFLECTION: Are you doubting yourself OR are you self-confident?

____

____

____

____

____

____

Chapter 2

Love, Relationships, Vitiligo…

Love yourself, and loving others will be the reason your life is

successful

~Cynthia K. Robertson

The most important thing to remember is that we must always love ourselves *first*. As we develop relationships there are those that truly see us as individuals… without blemishes or differences. In their eyes we are no different than they are. However, there are those who seemingly cannot accept people who differ from them physically, mentally, politically, financially and/or religiously. Fortunately, we dictate the relationships we develop… and if we love ourselves *first,* typically we choose our relationships wisely.

Everyone has personal biases that may inhibit their personal growth with a person seen as different by societal standards. This will make it difficult for relationships to blossom in their lives purposely. When people can't accept and be comfortable with other people's differences, their personal relationship will be thwarted.

Having Vitiligo while establishing personal relationships produces an array of emotions, challenges, and questions. Fortunately, some of us with Vitiligo have found that special person who is honest, transparent, affirming, and loving. The blessing of true love is a rarity, especially today! Life constantly presents unpredictable ups and downs, but love is the bond that makes life worth living.

I found my soulmate in 1985 and we were married for 34 years until he went home to be with the Lord. We shared an amazing journey as husband and wife, parents, and life partners. Undoubtedly, having a partner that understood and accepted that I had vitiligo… afforded me enhanced happiness and a sense of wellbeing that many in this world may never experience. For this, I am grateful.

My husband never questioned my appearance. As a matter of fact, I had to ask him! "Does my appearance bother you?" Emphatically, he stated, "NO, I will never LEAVE you or DENY you because of your appearance. I fell in love with you – NOT your skin. My husband's unconditional acceptance of ME helped me to EMBRACE all that I am *even* more!

Undoubtedly, there are those who don't understand skin disorders, their origin, and how it affects relationships. As a person with vitiligo (or any other condition that alters one's appearance), REAL questions and concerns must be addressed… Am I the *right* person for them? Will they be able to handle the questions, dubious looks, and possible rejection (of the relationship) from their family members and friends? If concerns like these aren't addressed the relationship will falter.

Having a strong sense of self-esteem, self-worth and knowing *who* we are and *whose* we are will take us further than we imagine. We ARE unique, magnificent and the world is OURS! Therefore, we can accomplish anything WE choose.

Undeniably, having purposeful and fulfilling relationships will allow us to GROW into the absolute BEST version of ourselves. So, be intentional about loving and accepting yourself and loving and accepting others *should* happen naturally.

However, I understand self-acceptance is NOT easy for those who have highly visible *imperfections*. Vitiligo has been a part of my identity since I was seven years old. Thankfully, my village embraced and loved me continually and their acceptance of me helped me accept myself!

Consider this, if your appearance is the only thing that is STOPPING you from living your BEST life – you've given this aspect of who you are too much power! Gratefully, our ability to FULLY show up as our authentic selves is the MOST powerful thing we can do! When we embrace ALL of who we are personally and relationally – we also empower others to do the same!

Reflect & Embrace It:

Reflection is a necessary practice for those who desire TO LOVE & EMBRACE themselves completely... DO this now, you're worth it!

In life you will encounter challenges and situations that make you question who you are. Only you can be consistent and reciprocate the true love you have for you! Don't expect others to embrace the life that has been created for you. Don't settle for less than you deserve. If you question your life, "don't".

REFLECTION: Are you EMRACING & LOVING yourself *first,* or do you seek love outside of yourself, first?

____

____

____

____

____

____

____

Chapter 3

I Am God's Masterpiece

Know and embrace your inner-beauty…
Baby you're God's Masterpiece.
~Cynthia K. Robertson

I have encountered several people of various nationalities that are unaware of cultural differences, not to mention dermatological differences. There are close to 2 million people from every ethnic background who have vitiligo. There are many who choose to cover their spots and discoloration with makeup to conceal their appearance.

While in college, I started concealing my spots. I did not want to answer questions regarding my appearance on a daily basis. I thought that it would distract me from moving forward successfully to reach my goal. The discoloration around my eyes, nose, fingers, and hands were perfectly visible to the world. However, I only concentrated on trying to mask the spots on my face.

There were several makeup concealers on the market, but most were not geared towards people of color (melanated skin). After researching, I found a concealer that matched my complexion almost perfectly. For a while, I loved the comfort the concealer seemingly provided… No unsolicited stares, glares, or insensitive questions.

Inevitably, there were several downsides to covering vitiligo. The cost was very expensive to maintain, the makeup couldn't adapt to the constant changes in my skin and the pattern of my vitiligo. The makeup always stained my clothing, sheets, pillowcases, and anything else my makeup came in contact with.

Although numerous new make ups and coverage for vitiligo were available to purchase, some of them were not FDA regulated at the time. Unfortunately, the side effects of using these weren't known until the damage was done.

One unforgettable morning the manner in which I saw myself changed! As I studied my reflection in my bathroom mirror, I said to myself "That's it…NO more makeup for me! I am a beautiful woman, and I will not hide what God intended for others to see… I am one of God's personal masterpieces!"

One day, while sitting in my office preparing for the day, a colleague I supervised knocked on the door and walked in. She looked at me and said, "Wow, you don't have on any makeup!" I happily responded, "No I'm not wearing makeup, and don't I look amazing!?!" We both smiled and she said, "You sure do!"

To this day, when I hear and see how blessed her life is, I remember how impactful her words of kindness were to my journey. Vonceil Levine-Jones, thank you for jumpstarting this turning point in my life. Knowing that I am a rare creation of God's beauty has allowed me to graciously EMBRACE and love ALL of me. I encourage each of you, to remind yourselves (daily) that you *too,* are one of God's masterpieces, I will embrace ME!

Reflect & Embrace It:

Reflection is a necessary practice for those who desire TO LOVE & EMBRACE themselves completely... DO this now, you're worth it!

You are unique, and NOTHING about who you were created to be replicated. This is a beautiful fact! So, on the days you FEEL like you're just NOT... Look, in the mirror and say, "I ABSOLUTELY AM...

REFLECTION: Embrace who you are, write it, and make it plain! Write at least 3 "I ABSOLUTELY AM affirmations:

____

____

____

____

____

____

____

Chapter 4

Vitiligo During Pregnancy...

My sons are blessings, being their mother is an honor.
~Cynthia K. Robertson

During both of my pregnancies, my autoimmune system changed substantially. My vitiligo accelerated and increased over my entire body. My dark skin became lighter and continually progressed. As the years went by my hands became lighter, new spots seemingly appeared overnight.

Honestly, my body was shocked! My Vitiligo patches on my face spread to my nose, ears, and mouth. Eventually it also spread to my fingers, arms and legs as well. The only change in my feet was the progression of pigment change from the top of my feet up towards my ankles.

My metamorphosis was gradual and noticeable. However, after a while I was no longer shocked by the changes, I saw day by day… and I welcomed them happily!

Although pregnancy increased the change in my physical appearance, I was not discontented at all! I have two amazing, strong, and intelligent sons who support me completely! They love me and my choice to love the skin I'm in.

My sons have not shown any signs of having Vitiligo nor have my granddaughters. Researchers have not confirmed that Vitiligo is hereditary. To further corroborate this finding, to my knowledge no one else in my family has a history of having vitiligo (just me –

because I am God's masterpiece).

33

Reflect & Embrace It:

Reflection is a necessary practice for those who desire TO LOVE & EMBRACE themselves completely… DO this now, you're worth it!

Our experiences are manifested blessings, because LIVING life to the fullest should not be taken for granted or forsaken! LIVE and EXPERIENCE life every day no matter what!

REFLECTION: Are you living life or is LIFE just happening to you:

____

____

____

____

____

____

____

____

Chapter 5

Health & Wellness with Vitiligo

Our health is the most valuable investment in which we have the ability to regulate ~Cynthia K. Robertson

As a person with vitiligo, I never imagined how this disorder could affect my body internally. Due to my deficient auto immune system, in 1999 I was diagnosed with hypertension and Type 1 diabetes with insulin dependency. Eventually, I was prescribed medicine to maintain a positive and functional health.

As a professional who worked long days and hours, while being a wife and mother to two athletic sons…I realized I needed to change my fast pace of life. I decided to become more active. So, I started attending Zumba and Step classes. Unfortunately, the negative progression of my medical condition happened quite rapidly.

In 2014, I *was* diagnosed with Stage 3 kidney failure. Again, I *attempted* to slow down. I continued exercising 5 days a week, but I had to stop soon after my diagnosis because I needed a kidney. My doctor informed me that my kidneys were failing and that I needed a transplant. I was placed on the kidney transplant list in Jacksonville, Florida at the Mayo Clinic. Irrefutably, this was an eye opener for me. I started dialysis in November of 2017, and I continued to work.

Research has shown due to a deficient immune system people with vitiligo usually have a second diagnosis which could be diabetes, inactive thyroid, lupus, and anemia to name a few. Well, I was anemic, had diabetes, and I've had my thyroid removed.

After being on dialysis for 6 months, I received a kidney transplant on June 18, 2018. God has truly blessed me throughout my life's journey! No matter what trials and tribulations I experienced… The final outcomes have been amazing (God had the last say-so)!

My health is great, my outlook on life is positive, and I refuse to *halfway* LOVE myself! I encourage everyone, even those without vitiligo, to exercise, maintain your health, and always seek medical advice and treatment for changes in your body that cause concern.

Yes, vitiligo can be a deal breaker (in some cases) but so can other life challenges and ailments. I am resolved in the fact that God created me perfectly. So, every chance you get to look in the mirror, I encourage you to remind yourself that you are beautiful and wonderfully made!

Reflect & Embrace It:

Reflection is a necessary practice for those who desire TO LOVE & EMBRACE themselves completely... DO this now, you're worth it!

Your life is one of the greatest gifts you will ever receive. Don't waste time on things and situations you have no control over. Be great, do great things and make your life matter.

REFLECTION: Greatness is a state of mind and being. Have you EMBRACED how GREAT you are?

____

____

____

____

____

____

____

____

____

Chapter 6

Skin in the Game *with* Vitiligo

Don't allow your ailments to STOP you, let them compel you to do what seems impossible! ~Cynthia K. Robertson

Currently, there still isn't a cure for Vitiligo. Maybe in the future, through medical science and research treatments will be developed to stop or slow down its progression. As of today, my entire body is 95% depigmented. My eyelashes, eyebrows, and skin are white.

When I admire my reflection (I never JUST look, there's a difference), I say, "Wow, God really LOVES me, my beauty is unique, and it cannot be replicated!" This is the essence of being created *wonderfully*!

I am excited, elated, and grateful that the world is moving in a positive direction regarding Vitiligo. I don't cover up my vitiligo nor am I self-conscious about my appearance. I am a member of several Vitiligo support groups which discuss new breakthroughs and give encouragement to those who feel they cannot EMBRACE their outer appearance.

I am also the administrator of my Vitiligo support group on Facebook. We are located in Gainesville, Florida for anyone who has vitiligo or wants to know about the latest treatments or has concerns about the disorder. The group is not just for those people who have vitiligo. We welcome friends, family members or anyone else who wants to be more informed about this disorder.

It is amazing to see that the world is finally embracing autoimmune disorders like vitiligo and publicly spotlighting models like Winnie Harlow. Thankfully, Vitiligo awareness is now becoming widespread throughout the world. However, even if people are cruel, uneducated, and insensitive regarding Vitiligo – don't allow their actions to deter YOU from living YOUR BEST life! EMBRACE your God-given uniqueness and know this - God didn't make any mistake when YOU were created! Embrace it!

JUST Embrace It:

EMBRACE YOU completely… DO this now, you're worth it!

REFLECTION: Embracing who we are is the GREATEST service to our CREATOR and OURSELVES. Nothing about who are is a mistake… God created US as masterpieces, adjust your confidence accordingly!

____

____

____

____

____

____

____

____

____

____

____

As I Look in the Mirror...

As I look in the mirror

Let me tell you what I see

An amazing strong person

Starring back at me

I proudly say to myself

How blessed God has been to me

I am so happy to be humble and set free

I love the way my eyes sparkle and shine

I love the way I laugh

I love the way I smile

I love being a good friend with a caring heart and mind

I always try not to frown

Never wanting to feel down

Knowing on this side of the world

I am blessed

Happy to be me and my vitiligo journey brings a glow to my face and a calmness to my heart.

I will always know that I am unique, special and a shade of color I can call my own.

I am…

Great

Unique

Beautiful

Wonderfully made!

About the Author

Cynthia K. Robertson, a retired Criminal Justice Professional, wife of the late Bobbie Robertson, mother, and now a nationally published author. She was born and raised in Gainesville, Florida and attended the University of Florida and Saint Leo University. Cynthia received a BA degree in Criminal Justice and a MS degree in Criminal Justice Administration. She is also member of the Gainesville Alumnae Chapter of Delta Sigma Theta Sorority Inc.

Cynthia's career afforded her the opportunity to look beyond the exterior of others and see the inner beauty that is sometimes hidden by the circumstances of life. In her debut literary work, "Embrace It: Loving Life with Vitiligo," Cynthia encourages her readers to love and accept themselves completely!

To connect and learn more about Cynthia Robertson, you can subscribe to her website at www.vitiligolove.com and follow her on all social media platforms.